This manual serves as an introduction to lymphedema therapy and to basic intervention techniques related to reducing edema. These techniques may be applied to a variety of clients with the cravats that we must monitor for changes and be aware that for every action there is a reaction.

The manual techniques presented should not be utilized on a client suffering from acute congestive heart failure, respiratory failure, or renal failure. Clients with a history of cardiac, respiratory, renal or circulatory compromise should be cleared for lymphedema therapy and edema management prior to initiating any lymphedema techniques. For optimal patient care, specific training with a lymphedema certified therapist and completion of lymphedema therapy certification is recommended.

This manual provides an introduction to lymphedema/edema therapy and will not provide specific information on compression wrapping and garments. The author recommends attending lymphedema therapy certification courses and additional educational training prior to utilizing compression wrapping and garments. Compression wrapping is a specific technique which requires training and close monitoring for client safety.

The information in this book is meant to supplement, not replace, proper lymphedema training and certification. Like any physical technique involving skin contact, these techniques pose some inherent risk. The authors and publisher advise readers to take full responsibility for safety by recognizing their personal skill and knowledge limitations. Before practicing the skills described in this manual, be sure that your client is aware of your training and level of expertise. Do not take risks beyond your level of experience, aptitude, training, and comfort level.

This book is not intended as a substitute for the medical advice of physicians or other healthcare providers. The reader should regularly consult a physician in matters relating to his/her client's health, and particularly with respect to any symptoms that may require diagnosis or medical attention.

This manual is dedicated to the caring professionals who make a difference in the lives of those with lymphedema.

A special thank you goes to Carmen Thompson who introduced me to lymphedema therapy and shared her clinical expertise. Carmen is making a difference by training professionals in the clinical management of lymphedema.

Special recognition is given for the contributions provided by Amanda Cross and the support offered by Radford University. With the Radford University's Graduate Research Fellowship grant, Amanda was able to participate in the editing phase of this manual in the spring of 2015.

Table of Contents

Introduction

Lymphedema therapy has gradually gained a foothold in the United States as a means to manage edema in clients with a variety of diagnoses. Initially, lymphedema therapy was associated with the treatment of edema for client's status post breast cancer, as lymph node removal often accompanied breast surgery. Recognition of lymphedema therapy interventions has expanded to include the treatment of edema associated with orthopedic surgeries and as a means to address the prevention of secondary complications caused by immobility and venous stasis. Wound care clinics are incorporating lymphedema therapy to assist with edema management of chronic wounds, venous and diabetic ulcers. The focus of lymphedema therapy, regardless of clinical setting, is to reduce and manage symptoms on a long term basis, as the related diagnosis is associated with irreversible changes to the lymphatic system (Yoshihiro, 2012).

This manual serves as an introduction to lymphedema therapy and to basic intervention techniques related to the management of non-pathological edema/lymphedema. By utilizing manual techniques, client education, therapeutic exercises and activities to treat edema and lymphedema, you are taking the first step in the journey of addressing the lymphatic care needs of your clients.

Definition of Edema/Lymphedema

Edema is defined as swelling that is caused by a surplus of fluid within bodily tissues. Although it can affect any part of the body, it most commonly occurs in the extremities (Mayo Clinic Staff, 2014).

Lymphedema is a condition in which excess protein-rich fluid collects in the interstitial space and surrounding tissue. Accumulation of lymphatic fluid can be due to damage or blockage of lymph nodes and vessels, as well as impaired venous return and elimination (Zuther, 2009).

Anatomy of the Lymphatic System

The lymphatic system lies parallel to the circulatory system, along visceral arteries and veins within the subcutaneous tissue. It is a low flow, passive system without an active pump; therefore, reliance is placed on the active pump of the venous system and muscle contractions, to return fluid that has accumulated in the interstitial space back to the circulatory system.

The human body is comprised of approximately 600-700 lymph nodes, located along the lymphatic vessels, acting as filtration systems for returning fluid. They are organized into clusters in the cervical, axillary, inguinal, pelvic, and thoracic regions. The abdomen contains the most lymph nodes (~200-300 nodes), followed by the groin area with approximately 50-70 nodes each, and the neck and axilla with ~ 30-50 nodes each (Zuther, 2009 & Foldi, 2003).

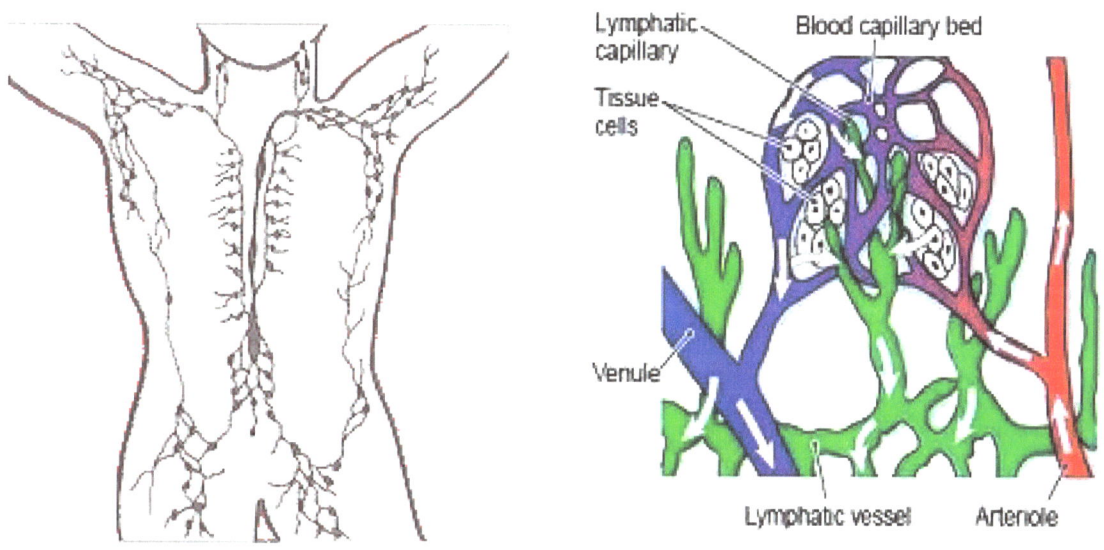

If the venous system is overloaded or distended, the venous valve mechanisms are unable to close and prevent back flow. Lymphatic vessels contain similar valve-like structures, and are loosely attached parallel to endothelial cells of blood capillaries. As fluid increases in the blood capillaries, lymph capillary cells easily separate allowing excess fluid to enter the lymph network and into the interstitial space. This fluid can accumulate and exceed the network's ability to move the fluid back into the circulatory system. This interstitial fluid accumulation leads to the development of **lymphedema** (Zuther, 2009). Gentle manual and compression techniques can be utilized to facilitate movement of this excess fluid into the circulatory system to allow elimination from the body (Zuther, 2009).

Under healthy conditions, lymphatic capillaries drain into collecting vessels containing valves to prevent backflow of lymph fluid. The lymphatic collecting vessels merge into regional draining pathways, called lymphatic trunks. The main regional lymphatic trunks are bilateral subclavian (located at the sternal notch), jugular, bronchomediastinal, and a single intestinal trunk. The regional lymph trunks drain into four lymphatic ducts. The lymph ducts then drain into the right and left subclavian veins. The thoracic duct drains the left side of body and right lower hemi-body, and the right thoracic duct drains the right upper body, thorax, and head (Zuther, 2009 & Foldi, 2003).

The target of treatment is the fragile lymph network lying just below the dermis layer of the skin. Therefore, feather light touch is required to avoid compressing the lymph network.

Functions of the Lymphatic System

Approximately 80% of fluid returned to the heart is accomplished by the venous system. The remaining 10-20%, along with any excess fluid, is returned by the lymphatic system (Zuther, 2009). The two systems work together to maintain blood flow, encourage tissue perfusion, and remove waste products. The lymphatic system specifically assists in returning interstitial proteins, water, and lipids to the bloodstream. Lymphatic fluid transports fats, waste materials, and lymphocytes, type of white blood cell (WBC), throughout the body (Zuther, 2009). The lymph fluid acts as a vehicle for WBCs, thus the lymphatic system is able to contribute to the body's immune response.

Lymph nodes serve to filter and thicken the lymph fluid, make lymphocytes, and store collected material which cannot be removed by the body such as coal, dust, and silica. Lymph nodes produce lymphocytes, which are the primary defense mechanisms against microorganisms and foreign materials collected before returning to the blood stream (Zuther, 2009 & Foldi, 2003).

Types of Lymphedema: Primary & Secondary Lymphedema

Although the etiology of primary lymphedema is unknown, the condition is most likely due to a malformation of the lymph vessels during fetal development. Primary lymphedema is considered to be an inherited disorder with approximately 1.15/100,000 diagnosed before age 20, with a related 4:1 ratio between affected women and men (Warren, 2007).

Secondary lymphedema is considered to be an acquired disorder, most commonly caused by invasive procedures such as surgery and radiation, and develops as a consequence of damage to the lymph vessels and nodes. It is estimated that there are 3 million new cases in the United States every year, including individuals diagnosed from the at risk population of documented venous insufficiency (Warren, 2007).

There are multiple causes of secondary lymphedema including cesarean section childbirth, cardiac bypass grafting, hip and knee replacement, and status post lymph node removal associated with neck surgery and cancer. Secondary lymphedema is often present following the development of stasis edema in dependent positioning and immobile persons (Suehiro et al., 2014). Diagnoses resulting in such dependence and immobility may include spinal cord injury, stroke, traumatic brain injury, cerebral palsy, and multiple sclerosis.

Following hip fracture repair or knee arthroscopy, many clients suffer with post-surgical edema/lymphedema hindering range of motion and mobility, potentially leading to secondary complications. Secondary complications may include superficial and deep vein thrombosis, tension and vascular wounds, and connective tissue contractures (scars). Non-ambulatory persons may suffer from stasis edema and develop cellulitis and wounds (Suehiro et al., 2014).

Lymphedema intervention is a critical prevention tool for therapists to consider adding to their skill set.

Staging of Lymphedema

Stages of Lymphedema	Description
Stage 0 	• Limited lymph transport capacity • No clinical evidence of edema • May have sensation of heaviness, ache, fatigue in the involved extremity
Stage 1 	• Accumulation of protein-rich, <u>soft-pitting</u> edema – which can be reversed through elevation (present on the lateral malleolus in the photo to the left) • Increases with activity, humidity, and heat
Stage 2 	• Accumulation of protein-rich, <u>non-pitting</u> edema due to presence of connective scar tissue • Presence of clinical fibrosis (present on the medial heel in the photo to the left) • Severe stage II, may notice skin changes: warts, eczema
Stage 3 	• Referred to as lymph-status/elephantiasis • Severe, non-pitting edema, fibrotic skin • Increase and accumulation of connective and scar tissue • Skin becomes thickened and leathery; development of folds and cracking of skin • Risk for yeast, fungi, and bacterial infections

Stages of Lymphedema table created with information gathered from Zuther, J.E. (2009). *Lymphedema management* (2nd ed.). New York, NY: Thieme Medical Publishers. Pictures provided by author unless otherwise noted.

Assessment of Lymphedema

The pitting edema scale is an easy to use objective measure of edema/lymphedema.

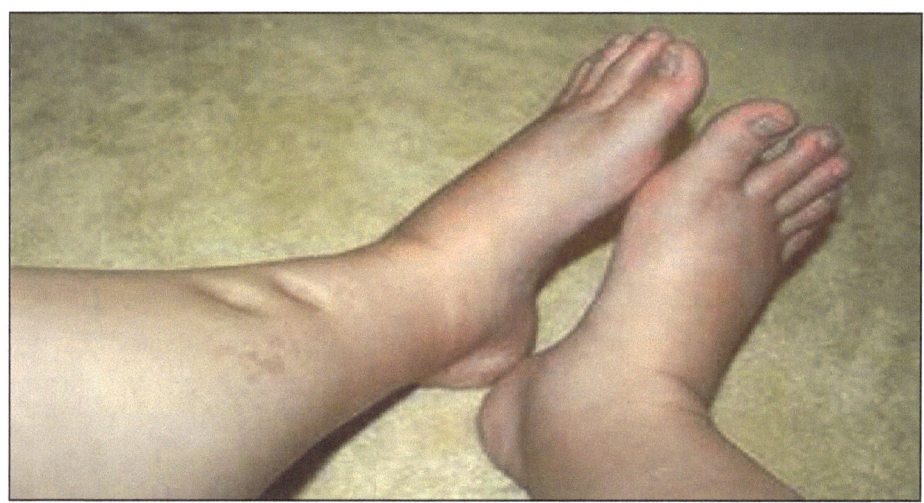

Scale	Description
1+	Barely detectable impression when finger is pressed into skin
2+	Slight indentation (15 seconds or less to rebound)
3+	Deeper indentation (up to 30 seconds to rebound)
4+	30 seconds or more to rebound

Edema Scale Table created from information provided by the Pitting Edema Scale: O'Sullivan, S.B. & Schmitz, T.J. (2007). *Physical rehabilitation: assessment and treatment* (5th ed). Philadelphia: F. A. Davis Company, p.659.

Limb Measurements

Circumferential measurements at consistent landmarks are essential to reliable monitoring and assessment of progress throughout edema management (Sanders, 2011).

Arm landmarks: Knuckles (MCP), wrist styloid processes, largest section of forearm, elbow joint line, and largest section of upper arm

Leg landmarks: Metatarsal line, heel/malleoli, smallest section of ankle, largest section of calf, knee joint line, largest section of thigh

Example measurement method:

To measure the upper extremity, begin at the proximal tip of the ulnar styloid process, and measure the limb every 5 cm with a flexible tape measure. For measurement of the lower extremity, begin from the proximal tip of the lateral malleolus, and measure again every 10 cm (Standard of Care: Lymphedema, 2007).

Limb Volume Calculation

Percentage of change in limb volume: Document the circumferential measurements of the limb before each session, and consider the results prior to treatment interventions.

Measurements taken again after the intervention will be utilized to document edema reduction, as a percentage of change in volume to demonstrate progress with treatment.

<u>Change in volume %</u> = 100 – (sum of measurements after intervention/sum of measurements before intervention) x 100

Location	Before	After
Knuckles	14 cm	13.5 cm
Styloid	16 cm	15.1 cm
Forearm	22 cm	19.8 cm
Elbow joint	26 cm	23.5 cm
Upper arm	34 cm	29.2 cm
Total	**112 cm**	**101.1 cm**

Example calculation, using values from the table provided:

Percentage change in limb volume
= 100 – (**101.1 cm / 112cm**) x 100
= 100 – [(**0.90**) x 100]
= 100 – 90
= 10

Change in limb volume = 10 %

Remember to include a functional link to the reduction in volume.
A client with a 10% reduction in limb volume will demonstrate an associated improvement in activities of daily living and mobility skills. Improvements in functional activities should be documented to accompany circumferential measurements taken during each visit.

Example Goal:
Client will demonstrate a 10% right arm volume reduction to allow increase use of upper extremities with activities of daily living (reaching in shower) within one week.

Other Signs and Symptoms of Lymphedema/Edema

Aside from swelling and fibrosis, the following may also be present upon initial examination:

- Skin changes: dryness, scaliness, cracking
- Altered sensation, numbness
- Impairments in strength and functional abilities
- Pain, aches, heaviness
- Fatigue
- Psychological issues associated with appearance:

The psychological consequences of lymphedema can be enormous for clients. As difficulty with functional mobility due to lymphedema increases, loss of independence, risk of incontinence due to immobility, and consequential decreased social interactions can be profound.

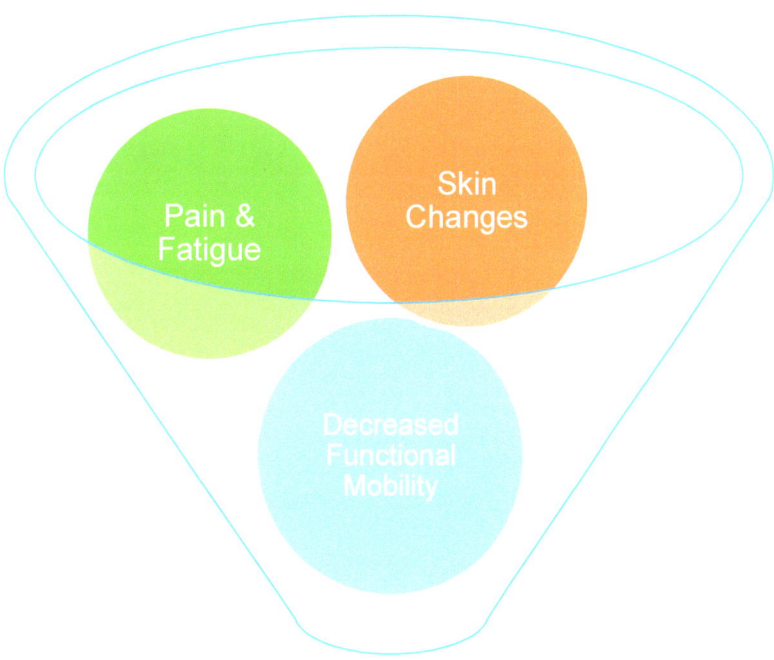

Psychological Distress

Related Diagnosis

Lipedema is the result of a disorder of lymph system formation during fetal development. The malformed lymph system develops corkscrew formations which trap deposits of subcutaneous adipose tissue. Individuals with lipedema present with bilateral swelling from hips to malleoli. Contrary to the usual lymphedema presentation, feet are not affected. An individual with lipedema will appear with a large buttock shelve and a relatively small portioned upper quadrant (picture). Losing weight does not change the bilateral lower quadrant and lower extremity presentation (Zuther, 2009 & Foldi, 2003).

Lipedema does respond to lymphedema therapy and compression. Without appropriate treatment, lymphedema may develop as a complication of the original lipedema diagnosis (Agbenorku, 2014).

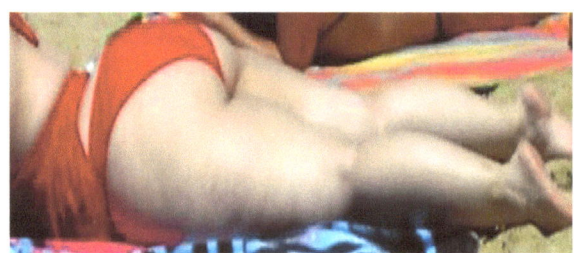

Contraindications for Lymphedema/Edema Therapy Techniques

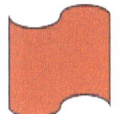 If the circulatory system is compromised and overloaded, congestive heart failure may occur or be exacerbated after lymphedema therapy as the body is unable to remove the excess fluid (Foldi, 2003).

Any signs or symptoms related to acute congestive heart failure are to be considered an emergent situation and require immediate medical care. Signs and symptoms of acute heart failure may include shortness of breath, inability to complete a normal daily activity such as dressing due to fatigue, edema in multiple extremities and a wet cough. **Any sudden change in breathing is considered an emergent situation. The techniques presented in this manual are not to be utilized on a client with cardiac, respiratory, and/or renal compromise.**

Manual techniques to move fluid into the lymph and venous systems are contraindicated for the following conditions:

- Acute, sudden-onset edema of unknown etiology
- Acute onset of shortness of breath (before, during, or after treatment),during a bronchial asthma flare up
- Inability to form and speak a complete sentence, and/or hyperventilation
- Acute congestive heart failure, compromised cardiopulmonary system, angina, uncontrolled or poorly managed hypertension
- Current diagnosis of deep vein thrombosis (DVT), suspected DVT, or pulmonary embolism (PE)
- Acute renal failure; compromised renal system, current dialysis regimen
- Acute inflammation, infection, gout, or cellulitis with symptoms (fever, chills, red streaking). Treatment of lymphedema after antibiotic administration depends on the recommendations of referring health care provider.
- Untreated cancer(s)
- Active bleeding (internal or external)
- History of aortic aneurysm or arterial insufficiency
- Severe arterial disease [peripheral artery disease (PAD), defined by ankle brachial index (ABI) of <0.5]
- Recent healing skin; at risk for re-injury
- Carotid stenosis or thyroid disorder; no manual techniques over the neck area
- Menses; avoid abdominal area as there is active bleeding present
- Medications; especially chemotherapy agents, have body dose residual times and must remain in the body (undisturbed) for a prescribed period of time. Lymphedema therapy techniques are not recommended while receiving chemotherapy. Consult the referring healthcare provider, and beware of all your client's medications (Zuther, 2009 & Foldi, 2003).

Professional judgment, client presentation and medical history will necessitate the need to determine the appropriateness of lymphedema techniques.

Considerations related to contraindications: Edema related to a trauma, significant orthopedic procedure, or systemic edema will require medical clearance and a referral to a certified lymphedema therapist (Manual Lymph Drainage/Completed Decongestive Physiotherapy).

Lymphedema Therapy / Edema Management Treatment

There is no cure for lymphedema. Lymphedema is a life-long condition which requires significant client education and training. Clients with lymphedema benefit from interventions addressing skin care, fluid drainage, exercises, and compression with the emphasis on self-management. Currently the primary treatment for lymphedema is Complete Decongestive Therapy (CDT). CDT is considered the gold standard of care for lymphedema (Mayrovitz, 2009 & Szuba 2000). The goal of CDT is to reduce the edema and achieve a stable state relative to each individual's medical condition and level of health. Self-management with a home maintenance plan is implemented during CDT to facilitate lifelong avoidance of future lymphedema progression (Szolnoky, 2014). Exacerbations of lymphedema may occur due to a variety of triggers such as bug bites, travel, and change in medications. Client education is a corner stone of CDT.

Elements of a CDT/ Lymphedema Therapy

- ➢ **Vitals**: including shortness of breath, and document health and history
- ➢ **Skin checks and circumferential edema measurements**
- ➢ **Manual techniques**
- ➢ **Therapeutic exercises**, activities, and functional mobility skills
- ➢ **Compression wrapping** - as appropriate *
- ➢ **Education**: specific to the client's lifestyle and treatment
- ➢ **Review self-management techniques**: self-stroking techniques, elevation, home exercises, skin care

*This manual provides select interventions to assist with the management of edema/lymphedema. The manual does not provide specific information on compression wrapping and garments. The author recommends pursuing lymphedema therapy certification and additional educational training prior to utilizing compression wrapping and garments. Compression wrapping is a specific technique which requires training and close monitoring for client safety.

Perform techniques with one extremity per session to determine tolerance to therapy. Monitor for shortness of breath. After manual techniques, have your client move the extremity, and perform exercises and therapeutic activities.

Traditional manual techniques are only one aspect to lymphedema therapy treatment, and are designed to be very light and gentle. Only superficial skin is moved to stimulate the underlying lymph network. Lymphedema drainage can occur, with the addition of deep abdominal breathing and regional node group stimulation. Deep manual techniques can be used to stimulate organs and deeper structures, but will not be discussed in this introductory text.

Recent research has identified Complete Decongestive Therapy (CDT) as the standard of care for treatment of lymphedema. This practice includes the implementation of manual lymph drainage, multilayer/short-stretch compression bandaging, gentle exercise, careful skin care, self-management education, and elastic compression garments (Evidence into Practice, 2015). **Each of the above interventions must be performed to be considered CDT.**

Phase 1 of CDT is usually performed 5 days/week depending on client's tolerance. The goal of this reductive phase is to decrease fluid volume of the limb until reaching a plateau. Frequency and duration should be individualized to each client, for optimal reduction in swelling and related symptoms (NLN Position Statement, 2011).

Phase 2 of CDT, otherwise known as the maintenance phase of CDT, should be implemented only at the point where the client demonstrates an ability to complete all aspects of Phase 1 independently. This requirement is important to maintain gains made in phase 1 of treatment. Treatment should still be altered as necessary, and any compression garments sent home with the client should be washed every 4-6 months (NLN Position Statement, 2011).

The light and gentle manual techniques utilized in manual lymph drainage, can assist with the reduction of lymphedema and should be performed in conjunction with exercises and therapeutic activities. Each of these interventions are stand-alone techniques and can be billed as skilled interventions such as manual therapy, therapeutic exercises, and activities, client/patient education, activities of daily living, and mobility training.

Simply performing manual techniques without therapeutic activities and exercises is **not** considered complete decongestive therapy or lymphedema therapy. All elements of CDT must be provided to bill as lymphedema therapy.

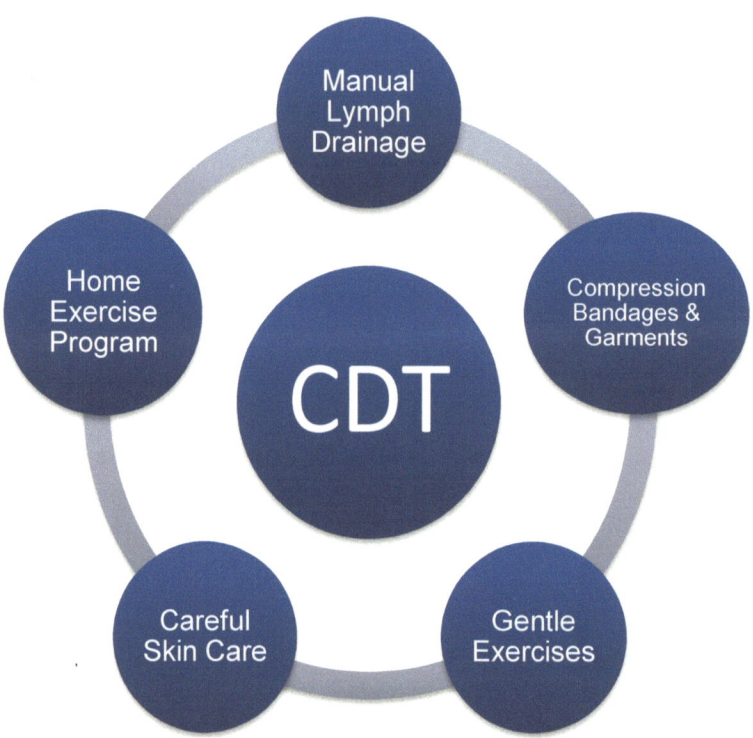

Compression bandaging is an integral aspect to CDT; however, as short stretch compression requires close monitoring and client supervision, the technique is not addressed in this manual. There are specific contraindications and precautions to consider before using compression bandages and/or garments for the treatment of lymphedema. Examples include arterial disease and/or ulcers, and signs of infection or wounds (Standard of Care: Lymphedema, 2007). If compression is applied incorrectly, patients may experience an increase in pain due to inappropriate tension, and subsequent decrease in circulation to the area being treated.

Successful application of compression bandages requires appropriate pressure, number of layers, components (such as addition of padding material), elasticity, and extensibility of the material used (Szolnoky, 2014). It is therefore recommended to attend certification training prior to compression application in the treatment of lymphedema. Compression garments are custom fitted medical devices, to be fitted and applied by a trained professional or a company representative.

Pneumatic compression pumps are available to assist with lymphedema management. The compression pumps are primarily utilized for palliative care as the pumps only assist the movement of the water component from the interstitial, while leaving protein content behind (Zuther, 2009). The proteins will draw water back into the interstitial, resulting in a continuation of the edema cycle. Diuretics function in a similar manner and thus can become part of the cyclical nature of edema (Foldi, 2003).

As diuretics are prescriptive and often critical in the treatment of cardiac conditions, therapists are not to recommend the discontinuation of any medication. Refer any client concerns regarding medications to the client's healthcare/referring provider.

Lymphedema techniques are an integral part of the health care plan. The duration of lymphedema techniques and therapy sessions can range from 10 minutes to over an hour, depending on the client and size of the affected limb. Frequency and duration are dependent on the client's needs and tolerance to treatment.

Typically, most lymphedema clients in outpatient practice settings are seen for an average of 6 visits, 2X per week. Prior to discharge from therapy, clients should be able to demonstrate full independence with each component of their prescribed home exercise program, to ensure maintenance of improvements made during treatment (Cohen, 2011). Therapy should comprehensively address mobility, strength, range of motion (ROM), flexibility, and as edema management.

Lymphedema therapy techniques have been shown in clinical practice to be effective in reducing edema and dramatically improving ROM, mobility, and wound healing within as little as 2 sessions. Lymphedema therapy techniques can be utilized for a variety of clients and diagnoses (Lasinski, 2012). Once the lymphedema is consistently managed, secondary complications from swollen, weeping skin, wounds, and venous stasis may be prevented.

This manual provides select interventions to address edema/lymphedema. Each of these interventions are stand-alone techniques and can be billed as skilled interventions such as manual therapy, therapeutic exercises, and activities, client/patient education, activities of daily living, and mobility training. These select techniques assist in managing edema and lymphedema. As compression wrapping is not instructed, these techniques cannot be billed as lymphedema therapy.

Lymphedema Therapy/Edema Management: Education & Prevention

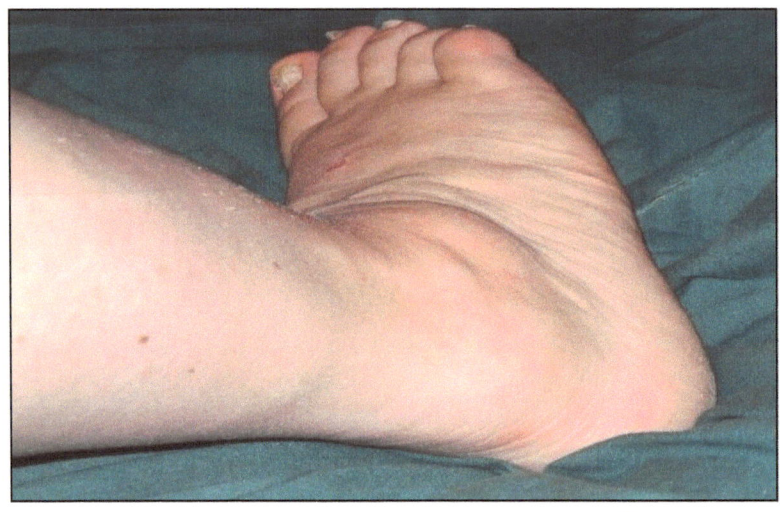

- ➤ **Skin Care:** Keep skin clean and dry; avoid use of fragrances, use appropriate nail care, practice good hydration habits, and protect problem areas such as wounds

- ➤ **Prevention:** Beware of bug bites, cat scratches, wear protective clothing outdoors, and always wear proper footwear

- ➤ **Self-Management:** Elevate the extremity, utilize appropriate compression options, and maintain adequate nutrition, self-stroking

- ➤ **Exercises & Mobility:** Walk, perform active range of motion of the affected limb (recommended multiple times per day)

It is important to inform clients that exercise for the treatment of lymphedema should not cause pain, discomfort, or soreness and should be performed in a slow and controlled manner (Zuther, 2009). Clients must consistently demonstrate appropriate skin care, communication with the treating health care provider, and adherence to the prescribed home exercise program prior to discharge (Zuther, 2009). Health care providers can improve the likelihood of these behaviors by providing handouts, videos, and written descriptions of expectations, in addition to the instructions provided in the clinic.

Depending on past and present history, clients may need to monitor electrolytes and blood sugar, as lymphedema treatment will alter balance of fluid and electrolytes (Standard of Care: Lymphedema, 2007).

Preventing the development of lymphedema begins with maintenance of an appropriate body mass index (BMI). As body mass increases, lymph transport and capacity become uneven (Ruocco, 2002).

For those individuals at risk for developing lymphedema, it is important to also provide education on adequate footwear, along with toe and foot hygiene (Lasinski, 2013). These patients may also be instructed to avoid walking barefoot at any time, in order to decrease the risk of injury or infection.

Following lymph node dissection surgery, patients should avoid cuts, burns, intravenous injections, and blood pressure measurements on the affected side (Prevention of secondary lymphedema, 2002). Hot tubs, high humidity, chronic venous insufficiency, and immobility are each potential triggering factors to the development or recurrence of lymphedema (Zuther, 2009).

Lymphedema/Edema Management: Basic Manual Techniques

Non-pathological lymphedema/edema management of Stage 1 and 2 Lymphedema with an intact lymph network:

The techniques described below are intended as an introduction to basic lymph drainage techniques, and do not address lymph drainage status post lymph node removal or major surgery resulting in disruption of the lymph and circulatory systems. The following techniques are intended for use with minor orthopedic surgeries, stasis edema, and as a means to address the prevention of secondary complications caused by immobility and venous stasis. If a client has sustained significant circulatory and lymphatic system disruption, they should be evaluated by their healthcare provider and a certified lymphedema therapist.

Perform one extremity at a time/session to determine the client's tolerance to therapy, and monitor for shortness of breath. After manual techniques, have your client move the extremity, perform exercise and therapeutic activities.

The Goal is for the lymph drainage to flow towards the regional lymph nodes.

> ➤ To achieve adequate lymph drainage, the pathway to the venous system must be cleared by stimulation of the abdominal lymph network with deep abdominal breathing. Deep abdominal breathing is achieved by cueing your client to breathe deeply and extend the abdominal wall. Phrases such as "make a belly" or "push your belly out" may be helpful. Placing your hand on your client's abdomen and cueing to "push my hand up" may also assist in achieving adequate deep abdominal breathing.
> ➤ The next step is stimulation of the nearest proximal regional lymph node grouping.
> ➤ Then, manual drainage techniques are performed, following steps 2-4 listed in the sequence below.
> ➤ Followed by active movement with deep breathing, range of motion, mobility such as walking, and functional tasks.

Rule of 5: Five repetitions for each technique (belly breathing & stimulations)
Five repetitions minimum for each stroke
Five second end range skin holds at the end of each stroke

Sequence:
1. Deep abdominal (belly) breathing to stimulate the deeper lymph network to assist initiation of the vacuum system for lymphatic flow (Gautam, 2011)
2. Regional lymph node grouping stimulation (5 circles/strokes in a gentle cyclic action, avoiding squeezing the lymph nodes groups)
3. Light manual stroking towards regional lymph node grouping (stroke direction is distal to proximal). The key is to remember gentle skin stretch/ light touch. Too much pressure will close the lymph vessels. Hold end range of skin stretch for the count of five.
4. Hand placements follow a proximal to distal path with stroke direction moving distal to proximal in first pass. Return back up the extremity with distal to proximal hand placements. Stretch stroke remains towards the regional lymph node grouping.
5. Deep abdominal breathing repeated.
6. Active movement of the treated extremity to assist lymph flow and fluid return to the venous system. (Foldi, 2003)

Perform on one extremity at a time to determine the client's tolerance to therapy, and to monitor for any adverse reactions. After the manual techniques, have your client move the extremity, perform exercises and therapeutic activities.

KEY

🟩 = Abdominal lymph node grouping

🟨 = Clavicular lymph node grouping (proximal clavicular area at sternal notch)

🟦 = Axillary lymph node grouping

🟧 = Inguinal lymph node grouping

Upper extremity key lymph groups: 🟩 🟨 🟦

Lower extremity key lymph groups: 🟩 🟨 🟧
Return to the venous system is
assisted with the inclusion of right clavicular grouping stimulation.

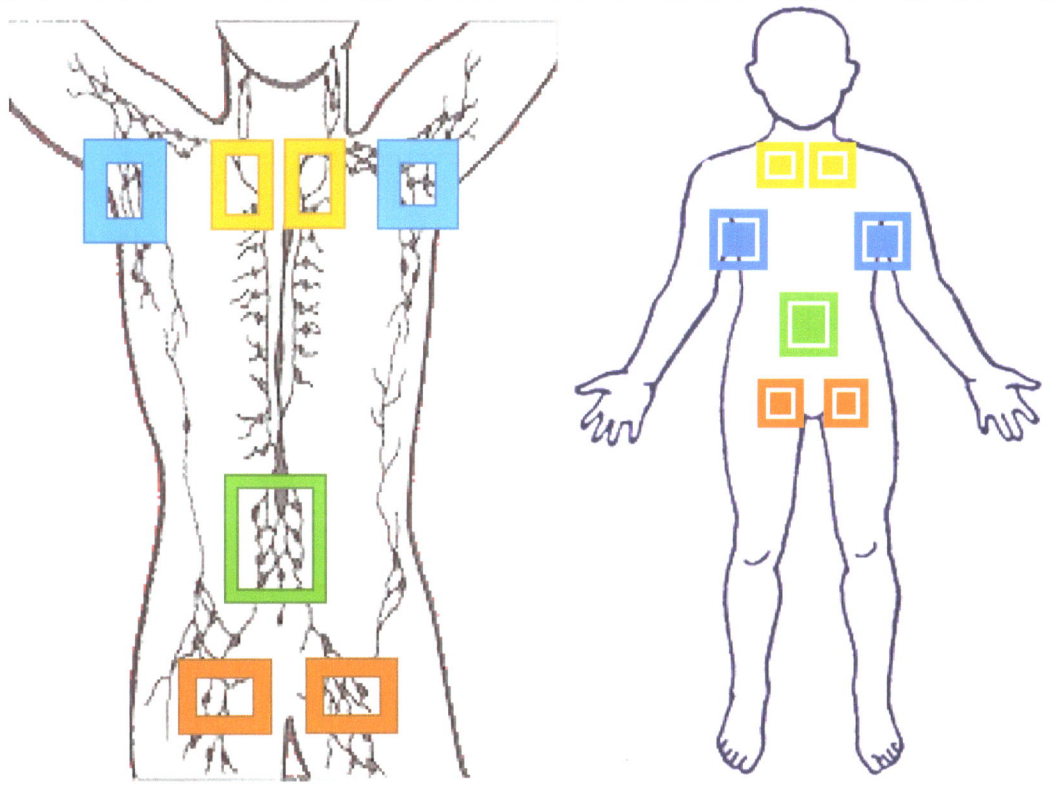

Feather-like gentle skin stretches ensure that the underlying lymph network is stimulated. If deeper pressure is applied, then the underlying lymph network is compressed. Compressed vessels will not be able to move the excess fluid, wastes and proteins from the interstitial space.

Hold each skin stretch position for the count of 5 (close to 5 seconds) and then release the stretch to allow the skin to return to a relaxed state. Do not slide your hand up and down the skin. Each stroke/skin stretch is moving towards the regional lymph nodes. The regional lymph nodes can then drain the excess fluid, wastes and proteins into the deeper lymph network system towards the renal clearance system.

The skin stretch stroke is <u>always</u> towards the regional lymph nodes.

Use the large surface contact area of your hands with each hand placement for node stimulation and along the extremities. Avoid digging finger tips and thumbs into the skin. The large contact area of whole hand will assist with gentle skin contact and lymph network stimulation.

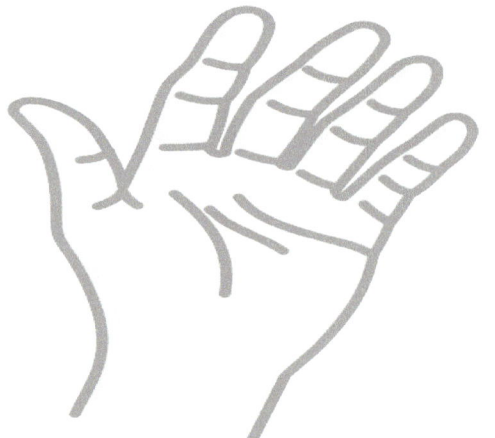 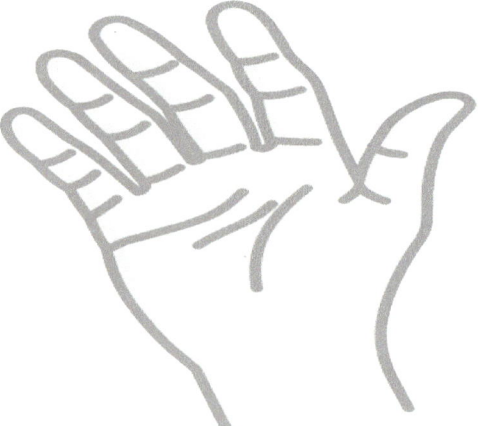

Upper Extremity Overview

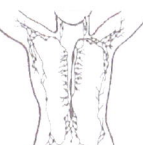

1. Deep belly breathing
2. Clavicular lymph node stimulation
3. Axillary lymph node stimulation

Stroke (skin stretch) direction will follow the arrows indicated on the arm, towards the regional lymph node group. ⬅

Hand placement will work in small increments along the extremity, from proximal to distal for the first pass then work back to the regional lymph node group.

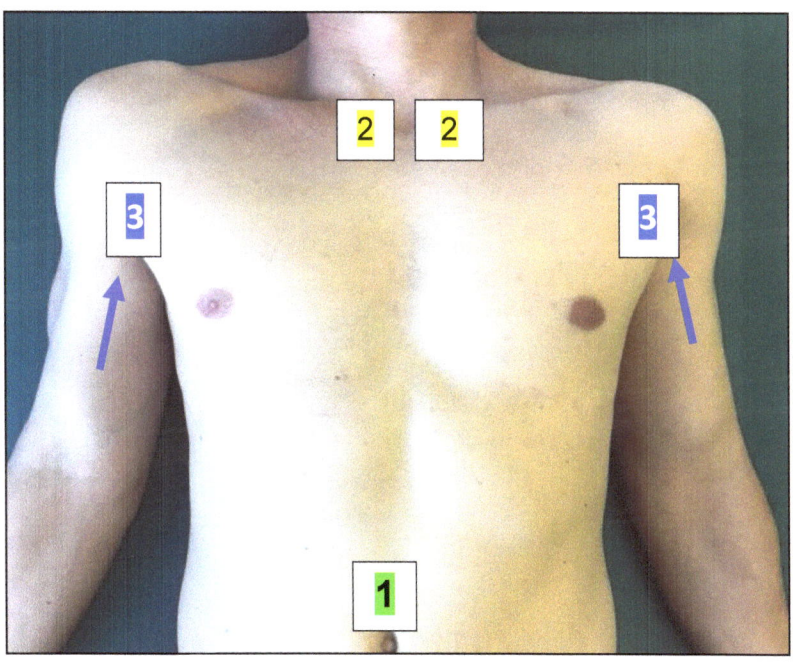

The following sequence flow illustrates the edema management manual techniques of an intact lymph network:

Upper Extremity:

1. Deep abdominal breathing X5

2. Clavicular lymph node grouping stimulation: pulsed circles X5

3. Axillary lymph node grouping stimulation: pulsed circles X5
Hand placement and stroke direction at axilla/shoulder is toward the sternum

4. Stroke direction is held for the count of 5 before releasing the skin and moving hand placement to the next position

5. Hand placement moves down the arm in short distance intervals; however, the stroke direction is towards the axilla

6. Hand placement continues distally to the hand/fingers with maintenance of stroke direction towards the axilla

7. Once reach most distal area, the second pass begins. Hand placement works back towards the axilla, slowly moving up the arm in short distance intervals with the stroke direction towards the axilla

8. Upon return to the axilla, gentle stimulation of the axillary lymph node grouping is performed with pulsed circles X5

9. Cervical lymph node grouping stimulation X5

10. Deep abdominal breathing X5

The skin stretch Stroke is <u>always</u> towards the regional lymph nodes.

Maintain a feather-like touch throughout treatment while stretching the skin towards the regional lymph nodes.

After Deep Belly Breathing, stimulate the regional lymph nodes.

Gentle circular press and release motions over the regional lymph nodes (Clavicular then axillary areas) for the count of 5

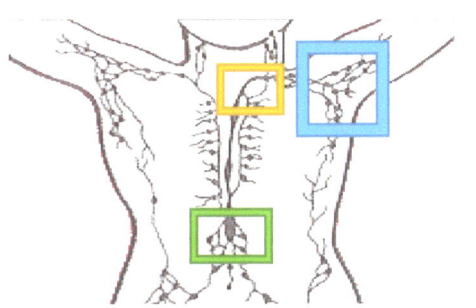

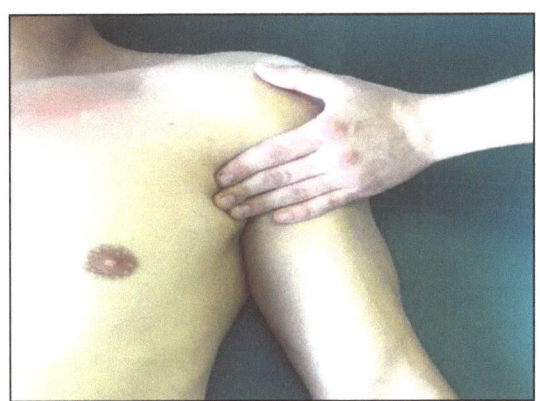

First hand placement following axillary lymph node stimulation is the most proximal on the extremity

Hand Placement:
1st sequence of hand placements, followed by second pass as described below:

Axilla → humerus → elbow → forearm → wrist → hand and fingers, then fingers and hand → wrist → forearm → elbow → humerus → axilla

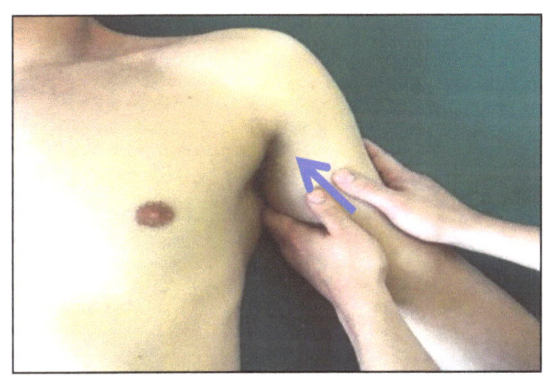

Remember the skin stretch Stroke is always towards the regional lymph nodes.

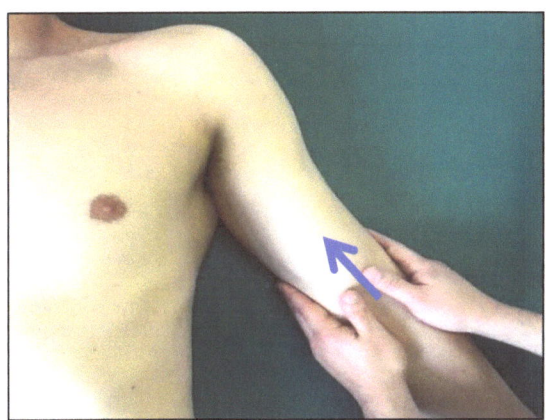

Lower Extremity:

1. Deep abdominal breathing X5

2. Groin/inguinal lymph node grouping stimulation: pulsed circular motions with the flat aspect of all finger pads X5

3. Hand placement moves distally and the stroke direction at groin/inguinal/lateral femur area is toward the abdomen

4. Stretch stroke direction is held for the count of 5 before releasing the skin and moving hand placement to the next position

5. Hand placement moves down the leg in short distance intervals; however, stroke direction is towards the groin area

6. Hand placement continues distally down the leg and you may stop to stimulate popliteal lymph nodes behind the knee, and continue towards the foot. Stroke direction is towards the groin area.

7. Hand placement slowly works back up (second pass) the leg in short distance intervals with the stroke direction still towards the groin area.

8. Upon return to the groin/inguinal area, gently stimulate the groin/inguinal lymph network and right clavicular node grouping X5

9. Deep abdominal breathing X5

The skin stretch Stroke is <u>always</u> towards the regional lymph nodes.

Maintain a feather-like touch throughout treatment while stretching the skin towards the regional lymph nodes.

After Deep Belly Breathing, stimulate the regional inguinal lymph nodes.

Gentle circular press and release motions over the inguinal lymph nodes for the count of 5

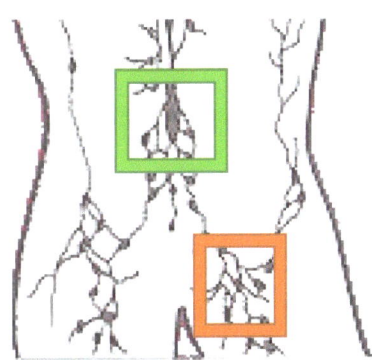

Hand Placement:

1st sequence of hand placements, followed by second pass as described below:

Thigh → knee → lower leg → ankle → foot and toes, then toes and foot → ankle→ lower leg → knee → thigh

Remember the Stroke is always towards the regional lymph nodes.

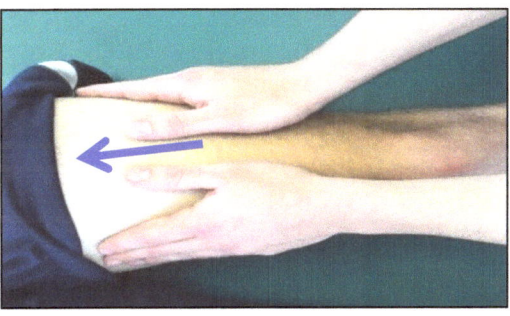

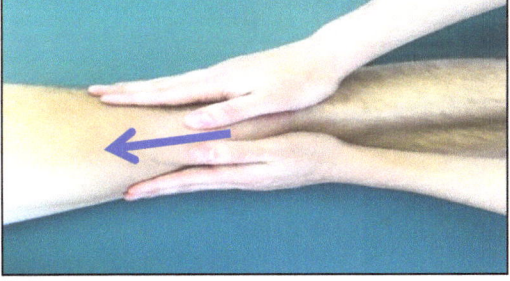

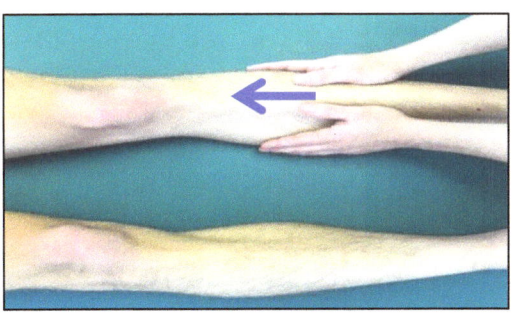

Lymphedema/Edema Therapy: Exercises

Types of Exercises

Movement facilitates lymph flow and venous return. Skeletal muscle contraction is the primary force in propelling lymphatic fluid throughout the system (Gautam, 2011). Encourage your clients to move. Include mobility and functional tasks with exercises and remember any movement is beneficial.

Sequencing of exercises will further assist lymph flow and venous return.

- Start at shoulder → elbow → wrist → hand, THEN movement of hand → wrist → elbow → shoulder
- Start at hip → knee → ankle → toes, THEN movement of toes → ankle → knee → hip
- Chair push-ups, walking, reaching and standing activities
- Deep breathing throughout exercises and activities will provide additional encouragement of lymph flow and venous return.
- Exercises can be performed in supine, sitting, and standing.

Example:

5-10 repetitions of knee raises (hip flexion), knee extension/flexion, ankle pumps, and toe crunches, THEN follow with toe crunches, ankle pumps, knee extension/flexion, and knee raises.

Edema Reduction Related Goal Examples

Upper Extremity Goals

- Client will demonstrate a 10% right arm volume reduction to allow an increase ease of upper extremity use with reaching within one week.
- Client will perform upper body dressing independently within two weeks.

Lower Extremity Goals

- Client will demonstrate a 10% right leg volume reduction facilitating transfers and gait within one week.
- Client will transfer with minimal assistance within two weeks.

Clients often require short duration edema intervention; and therefore, specific goals for edema management are written for 1-4 weeks, depending on the client. A long term edema management planning is necessary to avoid recurrent edema in the potential presence of causal factors. Long term edema management may require compression stockings, medication changes, nutritional counselling, and activity/life style changes.

Additional Considerations

Undiagnosed medical conditions: Closely monitoring clients undergoing any intervention is recommended. Baseline vital screen for blood pressure, heart rate, respiratory rate, temperature, pain and skin integrity, as well as overall perceived health/wellness and mobility questions will provide baseline information. Observe for any changes such as shortness of breath or discomfort. Stop immediately if there are signs of deterioration of the client's condition, notify his/her physician, and assist in seeking medical attention.

Footwear: Clients often present wearing footwear that is causing skin irritation. Clients may need to consider modifying or changing footwear to protect their skin, while maintaining hygiene and safety.

Hardened fibrotic areas: Manual lymphatic techniques should be performed for a longer duration and with increased repetitions in the affected area. Taping and myofasical techniques may be included to break up connective tissue restrictions and scar tissue, depending on the skin integrity and the client's sensitivity.

Hygiene: Clients are often unable to adequately perform daily hygiene. This can be related to obesity, adipose tissue, and edema limiting range of motion and mobility. Respectful discussions to include hygiene are an integral part of care.

Adipose compression:

During treatment of larger clients, adipose apron/pannus may compress the inguinal lymph nodes and contribute to lower extremity edema. Instruct the client to periodically lift the apron, in order to remove pressure from the inguinal area during exercises and manual techniques. Positioning in side-lying may also reduce the pressure.

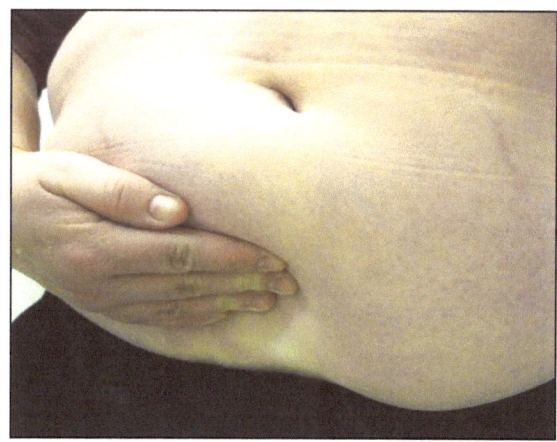

Infection: Venous stasis may occur in the presence of impaired circulation. This circulatory compromise may predispose clients to cellulitis, wounds, and infections. The extremity may be red due to venous stasis, indicating the need for close monitoring for other signs and symptoms of infection. These signs and symptoms may include: redness, warmth upon touch, fever, drainage, red streaks, malaise, and skin changes. Refer as appropriate

Personal safety: Weeping legs, wounds, and fungal infections may be present. Wear gloves and protect yourself as well as your clients by maintaining a healthy and clean environment.

Psychological impact of lymphedema: Lymphedema can be disfiguring and may hinder mobility and independence, causing associated social isolation and depression. Monitor and support your clients and refer to other providers as appropriate.

References

Agbenorku, P. (2014). Lymphedema: complications and management. *Surgical Science, 5*, 290-298. doi: 10.4236/ss.2014.57049

Cohen, M. (2011). Complete decongestive physical therapy in a patient with secondary lymphedema due to orthopedic trauma and surgery of the lower extremity. *Journal of the American Physical Therapy Association, 91*(11), 1618-1626. doi:10.2522/ptj.20100101

Foldi, M., & Strobenreuther, R. (2003). *Foundations of manual lymph drainage* (3rd ed.). St Louis, Missouri: Elsevier Mosby.

Gautam, A., Maiya, A., & Vidyasagar, M. (2011). Effect of home-based exercise program on lymphedema and quality of life in female post mastectomy patients: Pre-post intervention study. *Journal of Rehabilitation Research & Development, 48*(10), 1261-1268. doi:10.1682/JRRD.2010.05.0089

International Society of Lymphology. (2013). The diagnosis and treatment of peripheral lymphedema: 2013 Consensus document of the international society of lymphology. *Lymphology, 46*(1), 1-11. Retrieved from http://www.u.arizona.edu/~witte/2013consensus.pdf

Lasinski, B.B., McKillip, T.K., Squire, D., Austin, M.K., Smith, K.M., Wanchai, A., Green, J.M., Stewart, B.R., Cormier, J. N., & Armer, J.M. (2012). A systematic review of the evidence for complete decongestive therapy in the treatment of lymphedema from 2004 to 2011. *American Journal of Physical Medicine and Rehabilitation, 4*(8), 580-601. doi: 10.1016/j.pmrj.2012.05.003

Lasinski, B. (2013). Complete decongestive therapy for treatment of lymphedema. *Seminars in Oncology Nursing.* 29(1), 20-27. Retrieved from http://www.seminarsoncologynursing.com/article/S0749-2081%2812%2900083-6/pdf

Mayo Clinic Staff. (2014, September 6). *Diseases and conditions: Edema.* Retrieved April 20, 2015 from http://www.mayoclinic.org/diseases-conditions/edema/basics/definition/con-20033037

Mayrovitz, H.N. (2009). The standard of care for lymphedema: Current concepts and physiological considerations. *Lymphatic Research and Biology, 7,* 101-108. doi: 10.1089/lrb.2009.0006

Ogawa, Y. (2012). Recent advances in medical treatment for lymphedema. *Annals of Vascular Diseases, 5*(2), 139-144. doi: 10.3400/avd.ra.12.00006

O'Sullivan, S.B. & Schmitz, T.J. (2007). *Physical rehabilitation: Assessment and treatment* (5th ed). Philadelphia, PA: F. A. Davis Company.

O'Sullivan, S.B., & Schmitz, T.J. (2013). *Physical rehabilitation: Assessment and treatment* (6th ed). Philadelphia, PA: F.A. Davis Company.

Ruocco, V., Schwartz, R.A., & Ruocco, E. (2002). Lymphedema: An immunologically vulnerable site for development of neoplasms. *Journal of the American Academy of Dermatology, 47*,124–7. doi: http://dx.doi.org/10.1067/mjd.2002.120909

Sanders, J.E., & Fatone, S., (2011). Residual limb volume change: Systematic review of measurement and management. *Journal of Rehabilitation Research and Development, 48* (8), 949-986. Retrieved from http://www.rehab.research.va.gov/jour/11/488/pdf/sanders488.pdf

Suehiro, K., Morikage, N., Murakami, M., Yamashita, O., Ueda, K., Samura, M., & Hamano, K. (2014). A study of leg edema in immobile patients. *Circulation Journal, 78*(7), 1733-1739. Retrieved from https://www.jstage.jst.go.jp/article/circj/78/7/78_CJ-13-1599/_pdf

Szolnoky, G., Dobozy, A., & Kemeny, L. (2014). Towards an effective

management of chronic lymphedema. *Clinics in Dermatology, 32*(5), 685-

691. doi:10.1016/j.clindermatol.2014.04.017

Szuba, A., Cooke, J.P., Yousuf, S. & Rockson, S.G. (2000) Decongestive

lymphatic therapy for patients with cancer-related or primary lymphedema.

The American Journal of Medicine, 109, 296-300. doi:

http://dx.doi.org/10.1016/S0002-9343(00)00503-9

The Brigham and Women's Hospital, Inc. Department of Rehabilitation Services.

(2007). *Standard of care: Lymphedema.* Retrieved from

http://www.brighamandwomens.org/patients_visitors/pcs/rehabilitationserv

ices/physical%20therapy%20standards%20of%20care%20and%20protoc

ols/general%20-%20lymphedema.pdf

Warren, A.G., Brorson, H., Borud, L.I., & Slavin, S.A. (2007). Lymphedema: a

comprehensive review. *Annals of Plastic Surgery, 59*(4), 464-472.

Retrieved from

http://www.google.com/url?sa=t&rct=j&q=&esrc=s&source=web&cd=3&ve

d=0CDIQFjAC&url=http%3A%2F%2Fwww.researchgate.net%2Fprofile%2

FHakan_Brorson%2Fpublication%2F5942525_Lymphedema_a_compreh

ensive_review%2Flinks%2F0c960518fb98a4acf2000000.pdf&ei=dKE-

VaFcx8i1BeX5gdAl&usg=AFQjCNG0TfFDUNwz1Tl5a2ud7dDzNRkuPg&s

ig2=0AgtCjzv8_fddgAS8xv8Qg&bvm=bv.91665533,d.b2w

Zuther, J.E. (2009). *Lymphedema management* (2nd ed.). New York, NY: Thieme

Medical Publishers.

Resources

Inner Body Anatomy Explorer: http://www.innerbody.com/image/lympov.html

MedlinePlus (http://www.nlm.nih.gov/medlineplus/ency/article/002247.htm) offers general information and videos related to the lymphatic system:
- http://www.nlm.nih.gov/medlineplus/ency/anatomyvideos/000084.htm
- http://www.nlm.nih.gov/medlineplus/ency/anatomyvideos/000083.htm

Lymphedema therapy and certification information:
- http://www.lymphoedema.org
- http://www.lymphedemahope.com
- http://www.lymphnet.org
- http://www.lighthouselymphedema.org
- http://www.lymphedematreatmentact.org
- https://www.youtube/HA3h2JcCIxA

<u>Correspondence</u>

Address all correspondence to **Julia Castleberry MS PT, DPT, CLT, GCS, NCS**
Email: jcastleberry1@aol.com.
(CLT: certified lymphedema therapist)

Information and partial sections of this manual have been published in the American Physical Therapy Association Neurology Section's Stroke Special Interest website as part of an educational article related to post stroke interventions (2014). Building the case for lymphedema therapy for the prevention of secondary complications after injury.
Access: http://www.neuropt.org/special-interest-groups/stroke/featured-articles

This manual provides a general overview to lymphedema therapy and basic manual techniques. This manual does not provide instruction on all elements of lymphedema therapy; and therefore, individual treatments described should not be billed as lymphedema therapy or complete decongestive therapy. This manual does not take the place of lymphedema training and certification. Recommend the reader to pursue lymphedema certification when considering the treatment of oncology clients, and the medically complex.

Techniques utilized at the reader's discretion. Authors are not responsible for injury or harm. Request permission to copy.

www.ingramcontent.com/pod-product-compliance
Lightning Source LLC
Chambersburg PA
CBHW050404180526
45159CB00005B/2151